GW00356874

miracle juices™
stress
busters

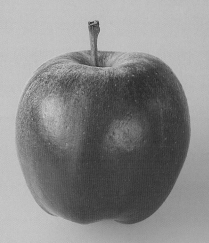

Safety Note

Stress Busters should not be considered a replacement for
professional medical treatment; a physician should be
consulted on all matters relating to health. While the advice and
information in this book is believed to be accurate, the publisher
cannot accept any legal responsibility or liability for any injury
or illness sustained while following the advice in this book.

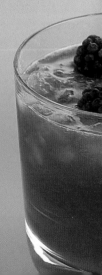

First published in Great Britain in 2002 by Hamlyn,
a division of Octopus Publishing Group Ltd
2–4 Heron Quays, London E14 4JP

ISBN 0 600 60671 6

A CIP catalogue record for this book is available
from the British Library

Printed and bound in China

10 9 8 7 6 5 4 3 2 1

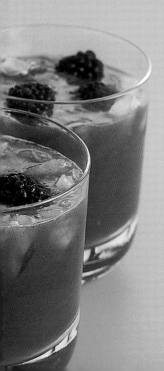

Contents

introduction

We all freely throw the word 'stress' about when describing how we feel, but how many of us fully understand its true nature and impact on the human body? For starters, stress isn't just the result of a late train or mounting pile of bills.

In the modern world we are constantly bombarded with all types of external and internal stress. Everything from the polluted air we breathe to the junk food we put into our systems can disturb the delicate balance our bodies are trying to maintain in order to function efficiently. Add to this a heavy workload, throw in a few emotional problems and, hey presto, you have a walking time bomb just waiting to explode.

The body's reaction to stress

How our bodies react to stress is rooted in our distant past. Early man would never have survived had it not been for the 'fight or flight' response to danger. When threatened, his adrenal glands would have pumped out increased amounts of the stress

Internal stresses
- Food allergies and intolerances
- Metabolic waste
- Chemical imbalances
- Nutritional deficiencies
- Blood sugar imbalances
- High cholesterol
- Auto-immune disease

External stresses
- Pollution
- Hydrogenated fats
- Smoking and alcohol
- Excessive UV exposure
- Heavy workload
- Emotional problems
- Bereavement
- Divorce or separation

hormones adrenalin and cortisol in order to step up his body's energy production. This would have raised his heart rate and blood pressure, increased the amount of glucose released into his blood by his liver, tensed his muscles, slowed his digestion, and thickened his blood in case of injury. We still react in the same way when we feel under stress. But unlike our early ancestors who expended all this extra energy by either running like hell or fighting, we tend to remain in a permanent state of heightened stress. This can keep hormone levels, blood pressure and the amount of glucose in the blood abnormally high. If this situation is prolonged the body accepts these levels as normal and adapts accordingly, with potentially dangerous effects.

Symptoms of excessive stress

- Chronic sore throat
- Urgency to urinate – adrenal glands and kidneys in trouble
- Palpitations
- Shallow breathing
- Short-tempered behaviour/mood swings
- Nervous twitching of eyelids
- Disturbed sleep patterns
- Anxiety
- Frequent colds and flu due to suppressed immune system
- Depression
- Skin irritation
- Food cravings
- Constant fatigue
- Loss of appetite and weight loss

5

food and stress

If your body is overstressed and feeling drained, the physiological effects of stress will be exacerbated by a poor diet. Unhealthy eating results in insufficient nutrients for the body and depleted energy levels. It can even result in food allergies and intolerances that cause further stress to the body by overworking the adrenal glands. This in turn produces an excess of the hormone cortisol, which leads to poor digestion and even inadequate thyroid function and the breakdown of muscle and bone tissue in the body.

The answer is to cut out all the foods that have a negative effect on your body, such as alcohol, caffeine and sugar – stimulants that interfere with adrenal function. You will also need to eradicate refined and processed foods from your diet, as these will put additional stress on your liver and digestive system.

Detox

The best possible de-stressing gift you could give yourself is a two- or three-day detoxifying break, ideally at the weekend when you have a chance to slow down. Make sure you

---

Top stress-busting foods

lettuce	dark green vegetables
bananas	chamomile tea
celery	cucumber
soya milk	watermelon
fennel	pineapple
sunflower seeds	parsley

have an abundance of fruits and vegetables (organic, if possible) at home. Eat and drink only raw food and drink loads of mineral water.

Aim to have three or four green vegetable juices per day and, if you drink fruit juices, then dilute them with water to reduce their sugar content. Eat one or two salads of raw vegetables, perhaps with a scattering of sunflower seeds. Exercise gently and get as much sleep as you can. Maybe try a little meditation or yoga.

If you get headaches or aches and pains during the detox, this is because your body is eliminating toxins, so focus on how good you are going to feel afterwards. Remember that stress is an individual experience; every person reacts differently. Try to change your perception of what stresses you and slow down the pace of your life sufficiently so that you have enough time for a healthy diet,

exercise and relaxation. 'Time out' is better than 'burn out'.

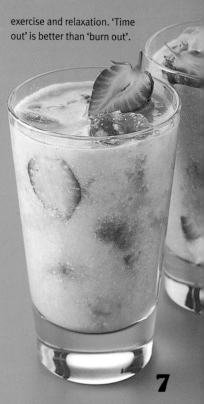

vital stress-busting nutrients

Nutrient	Actions	Good Source	Recommended Daily Dosage
Vitamin A	Vital for reducing susceptibility to infection by maintaining mucous membranes, antioxidant, essential for good digestion	Preformed Vitamin A found in milk, cheese, butter, eggs and all meats, fish liver oil. Beta-carotene found in yellow or deep orange fruits and vegetables such as cantaloupe, butternut squash, or dark leafy green vegetables such as spinach, broccoli and beet greens	5000 IU men 4000 IU women 2000 IU children
Vitamin B5	Supports normal functioning of adrenal glands, maintains healthy digestive and nervous system, vital to help body withstand stress	Brewer's yeast, sunflower seeds, blue cheese, corn, lentils, soybeans, whole grains, wheat germ, salmon, egg yolks, meat	10–15 mg is normal, although an adult could safely raise intake to 500 mg during stressful periods
Vitamin C	Powerful antioxidant, reduces allergic reactions, helps to form red blood cells, vital for healthy adrenal function	Citrus fruits, all black and red berries, papaya, tomatoes, kiwi fruits, broccoli, cantaloupe, red peppers, cabbage, mango	The absolute minimum is 60 mg, but during times of stress increase this to 1–2 g per day, divided into two doses
Vitamin E	Antioxidant, oxygenates the blood, thins the blood, lowers blood pressure	Cold pressed oils, eggs, wheat germ, molasses, sweet potatoes, leafy vegetables, sunflower seeds, nuts, cashews, soybeans, organ meats, avocados	An adult could safely take up to 600 IU daily

Nutrient	Actions	Good Source	Recommended Daily Dosage
Zinc	Protects immune system, aids digestion and helps the metabolism of proteins, fats and carbohydrates, helps to regulate blood sugar	Pumpkin seeds, sunflower seeds, seafood, mushrooms, brewer's yeast, soybeans, eggs, wheat germ, meat	12–15 mg
Selenium	Natural antioxidant, necessary for production of prostglandins, which affect blood pressure	Brewer's yeast, wheat germ, whole grains, sesame seeds, sunflower seeds, brazil nuts, seafood, cabbage, broccoli, cucumber, garlic, onions, radishes	50–200 mg
Magnesium	Primary mineral required by adrenal glands, helps absorption of vitamins, B, C and E, neurotransmission and activity	Green vegetables, wheat germ, soybeans, whole grains, seafood, figs, corn, apples, peaches, apricots, nuts, especially almonds	300–350 mg
Tryptophan	A natural relaxant, helps alleviate insomnia by inducing normal sleep; reduces anxiety and depression; helps in the treatment of migraines; boosts the immune system; reduces the risk of artery and heart spasms and works with lysine to lower cholesterol levels	Bananas, turkey, fish, avocados, seaweed, dark leafy green vegetables, potatoes, sunflower seeds, pumpkin, milk	200 mg

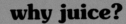

why juice?

Vital vitamins and minerals such as antioxidants, vitamins A, B, C and E, folic acid, potassium, calcium, magnesium, zinc and amino acids are present in fresh fruits and vegetables, and are all necessary for optimum health. Because juicing removes the indigestible fibre in fruits and vegetables, the nutrients are available to the body in much larger quantities than if the piece of fruit or vegetable were eaten whole. For example, when you eat a raw carrot you are able to assimilate only about 1 per cent of the available beta-carotene, because many of the nutrients are trapped in the fibre. When a carrot is juiced, thereby removing the fibre, nearly 100 per cent of the beta-carotene can be assimilated. Juicing several types of fruits and vegetables on a daily basis is therefore an easy way to ensure that your body receives its full quota of these vital vitamins and minerals.

In addition, fruits and vegetables provide another substance absolutely essential for good health — water. Most people don't consume enough water. In fact, many of the fluids we drink — coffee, tea, soft drinks, alcoholic beverages and artificially flavoured drinks — contain substances that require extra water for the body to eliminate, and tend to be dehydrating. Fruit and vegetable juices are free of these unnecessary substances.

Your health

A diet high in fruits and vegetables can prevent and help to cure a wide range of ailments. At the cutting edge of nutritional research are the plant chemicals known as phytochemicals, which hold the key to preventing deadly diseases such as cancer and heart disease, and others such as asthma, arthritis and allergies.

Although juicing benefits your overall health, it should be used only to complement your daily eating plan. You must still eat enough from the other food groups (such as grains, dairy food and pulses) to ensure your body maintains strong bones and healthy cells. If you are following a specially prescribed diet, or are under medical supervision, you should discuss any drastic changes with your health practitioner before beginning any type of new health regime.

how to juice

Available in a variety of models, juicers work by separating the fruit and vegetable juice from the pulp. Choose a juicer with a reputable brand name, that has an opening big enough for larger fruits and vegetables, and make sure it is easy to take apart and clean, otherwise you may become discouraged from using it.

Types of juicer

A citrus juicer or lemon squeezer is ideal for extracting the juice from oranges, lemons, limes and grapefruit, especially if you want to add just a small amount of citrus juice to another liquid. Pure citrus juice has a high acid content, which may upset your stomach, so it is best diluted.

Centrifugal juicers are the most widely used and affordable juicers available. Fresh fruits and vegetables are fed into a rapidly spinning grater, and the pulp separated from the juice by centrifugal force. The pulp is retained in the machine while the juice runs into a separate jug. A centrifugal juicer produces less juice than the more expensive masticating juicer, which works by pulverizing fruits and vegetables, and pushing them through a wire mesh with immense force.

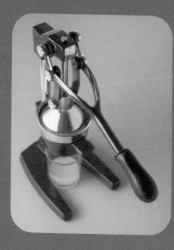

to two parts water will lessen any staining produced by the fruits and vegetables.

Preparing produce for juicing

It is best to prepare ingredients just before juicing so that fewer nutrients are lost through oxidization. Cut or tear foods into manageable pieces for juicing. If the ingredients are not organic, do not include stems, skins or roots, but if the produce is organic, you can put everything in the juicer. However, don't include the skins from pineapple, mango, papaya, citrus fruit and banana, and remove the stones from avocados, apricots, peaches, mangoes and plums. You can include melon seeds, particularly watermelon, as these are full of juice. For grape juice, choose green grapes with an amber tinge or black grapes with a darkish bloom. Leave the pith on lemons for the pectin content.

Cleaning the juicer

Clean your juicing machine thoroughly, as any residue left may harbour bacterial growth — a toothbrush or nailbrush works well for removing stubborn residual pulp. Leaving the equipment to soak in warm soapy water will loosen the residue from those hard-to-reach places. A solution made up of one part white vinegar

13

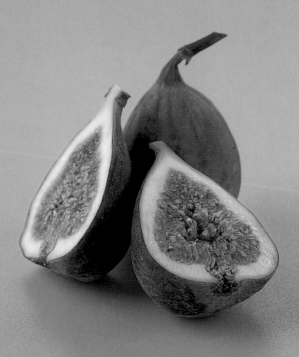

let off steam

As well as being very high in the immune-boosting vitamins A and C, this juice is fantastic for your digestive tract. The sweet potato removes any toxic build-up and will calm inflammation, and the carrots kill bacteria and viruses. So, if you are feeling the dual effects of burning the midnight oil and eating junk food on the run, this is the ideal juice to put you back on track.

back on track

150 g (5 oz) sweet potato
2 small oranges, peeled
150 g (5 oz) carrots

Juice the sweet potato, oranges and carrots. To make a smoother, creamier drink, transfer the juice to a blender and process with a couple of ice cubes. Decorate with mint sprigs, if liked.
Makes 200 ml (7 fl oz)

Nutritional values

- Kcals 358
- Carbohydrate 88 g
- Fat 2.1 g
- Vitamin A 78357 IU
- Vitamin C 200 mg

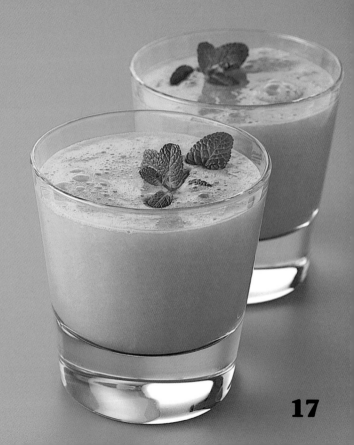

17

A natural tranquilizer, lettuce contains small amounts of lactucin, which is known to induce a state of relaxation. The apple, besides being packed full of nutrients, gives this juice a comforting natural sweetness.

tranquillizer

**175 g (6 oz) Romaine
lettuce
1 apple, about 250 g
(8 oz)**

Juice the lettuce and apple. Place ice cubes in a tall glass and pour the juice over them. Serve immediately, decorated with apple slices if liked.
Makes 200 ml (7 fl oz)

Nutritional values

- Kcals 71
- Carbohydrate 14 g
- Fat 1 g
- Vitamin C 21 mg
- Magnesium 52 mg
- Tryptophan 76 mg

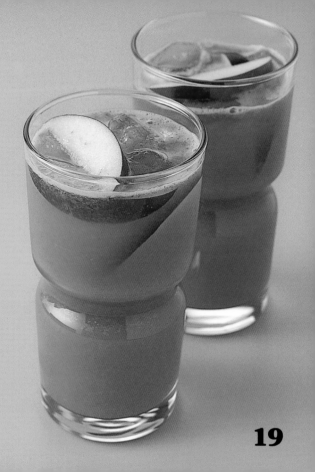

19

When you are stressed you will quite often find that your digestion and circulation are affected, leaving you feeling fatigued and lacking in energy. Red peppers are excellent for reducing blood pressure and papaya is renowned for its digestive properties.

deep breath

1 large tomato
100 g (3½ oz) red pepper, cored and deseeded
about 125 g (4 oz) papaya, skinned and deseeded

Juice the tomato, red pepper and papaya. Pour the juice into a blender, add a couple of ice cubes and process. Serve decorated with slivers of red pepper, if liked.

Makes 200 ml (7 fl oz)

Nutritional values

- Kcals 124
- Carbohydrate 21.5 g
- Fat 0.6 g
- Vitamin A 10851 IU
- Vitamin C 315 mg
- Magnesium 51 mg

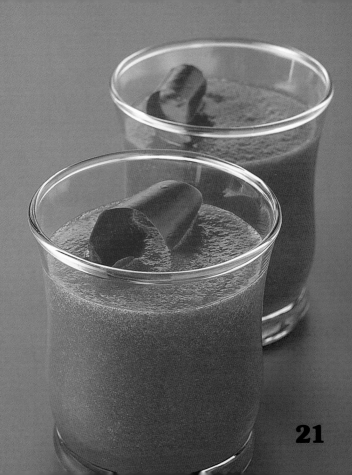

21

If you are getting wound up about something, take five minutes and chill out with this relaxing elixir. Fennel has antispasmodic properties and, when combined with naturally calming chamomile tea, this drink should settle even the most nervous of stomachs.

chill pill

**1 small fennel bulb,
about 150 g (5 oz)
1 lemon, peeled
100 ml (3½ fl oz) chilled
chamomile tea**

Juice the fennel and lemon, then mix with the chamomile tea. Serve over ice with some lemon slices, if liked.

Makes 200 ml (7 fl oz)

Nutritional values

- Kcals 55
- Carbohydrate 13 g
- Fat 0.3 g
- Vitamin C 33 mg
- Magnesium 25 mg

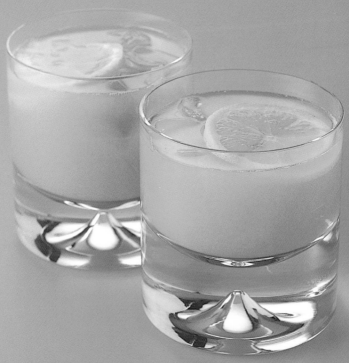

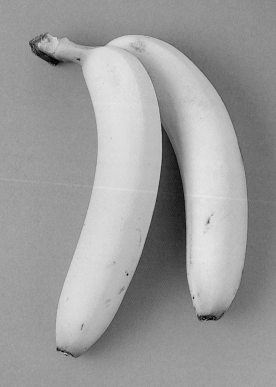

unwind

Pineapple contains bromelin, an enzyme that aids digestion and acts in a similar way to stomach acid. It is also believed to be highly effective at dissolving blood clots; its downside is that it is not very kind to tooth enamel and is therefore best drunk diluted. (Cleaning your teeth after consuming fresh pineapple is also a good idea.) Celery is the perfect accompaniment as it, too, aids digestion and lowers blood pressure. This juice is good for re-energizing, detoxifying the liver and replenishing lost fluids.

hi tension

**150 g (5 oz) pineapple
chunks
150 g (5 oz) celery
½ lemon, peeled**

Juice all the ingredients then serve over ice in a tall glass. Decorate with some sprigs of mint, if liked.
Makes 200 ml (7 fl oz)

Nutritional values

- Kcals 101
- Carbohydrate 27 g
- Fat 1.1 g
- Vitamin C 33 mg
- Magnesium 41 mg

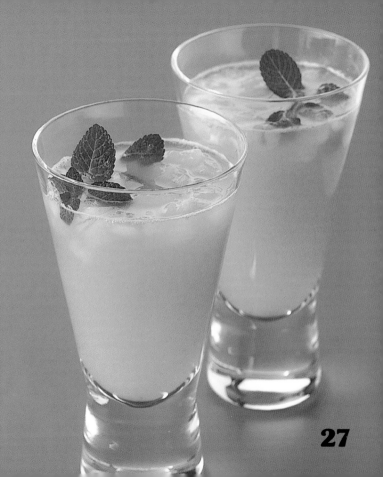

Lettuce contains a natural sedative called lactucin, which has been shown to have a calming effect on the mind and body. Grapes are effective at lowering blood pressure, so make this juice when you feel your pressure levels rising. It has a sharp taste with sweet undertones.

neuro zen

200 g (7 oz) white grapes
200 g (7 oz) lettuce
2.5 cm (1 inch) cube fresh root ginger, chopped

Juice all the ingredients. Serve over ice, or pour into a blender and process with ice cubes for a creamier drink. Decorate with grapes, if liked.

Makes 200 ml (7 fl oz)

Nutritional values

- Kcals 134
- Carbohydrate 31 g
- Fat 0.6 g
- Vitamin C 20 mg
- Selenium 0.8 mg
- Tryptophan 90 mg

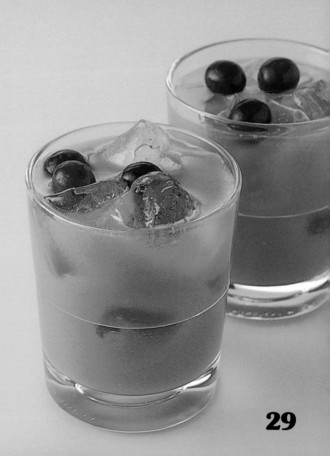

This cooling juice supplies almost a complete daily quota of beta-carotene, and the apples are superb for lowering blood cholesterol. Make sure you juice them with the pips, as the pectin is very effective at helping to remove any toxins that may be building up in your overworked system.

panic
attack

2 apples
3 apricots, halved and
stoned
1 peach, halved and
stoned

Juice the apples, apricots and peach. Pour into a blender with a few ice cubes and whizz for 10 seconds. Serve in a tall glass and decorate with peach slices, if liked.
Makes 200 ml (7 fl oz)

Nutritional values

- Kcals 238
- Carbohydrate 73 g
- Fat 1.5 g
- Vitamin A 3382 IU
- Vitamin C 32 mg
- Magnesium 26 mg

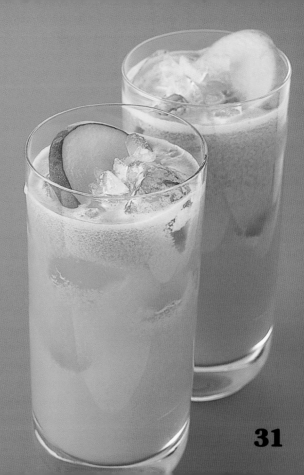

Since the magnesium in the parsley and celery has a calming effect, this juice is ideal when you feel pressured. Garlic is a marvellous all-round health-giving food, renowned for its antibacterial, antibiotic, antiseptic and antiviral properties.

rootiful

175 g (6 oz) carrot
175 g (6 oz) parsnip
175 g (6 oz) celery
175 g (6 oz) sweet potato
a handful of parsley
1 garlic clove

Juice all the ingredients together then whizz in a blender with a couple of ice cubes. Serve in a wide glass decorated with a wedge of lemon and a sprig of parsley, if liked.

Makes 200 ml (7 fl oz)

Nutritional values

- Kcals 386
- Carbohydrate 83 g
- Fat 0.9 g
- Vitamin A 51192 IU
- Vitamin C 136.35 mg
- Magnesium 150.5 mg

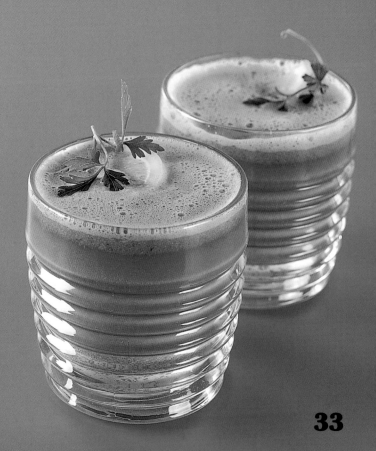

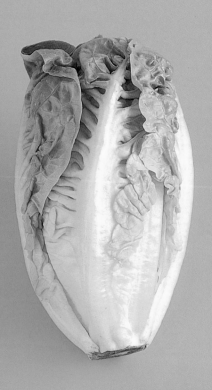

calm

All three ingredients in this juice are high in magnesium and vitamin C, which are essential for the healthy functioning of the adrenal glands and the liver. If you are going through a prolonged period of stress, the chances are that your body is lacking these two vital nutrients as they are easily depleted when the going gets tough.

stress buster

150 g (5 oz) spinach
150 g (5 oz) broccoli
2 tomatoes

Juice the spinach, broccoli and tomatoes. Serve in a tumbler over ice, decorated with sliced tomatoes, if liked.
Makes 200 ml (7 fl oz)

Nutritional values

- Kcals 120
- Carbohydrate 23 g
- Fat 1.5 g
- Vitamin A 14234 IU
- Vitamin C 202 mg
- Magnesium 171 mg

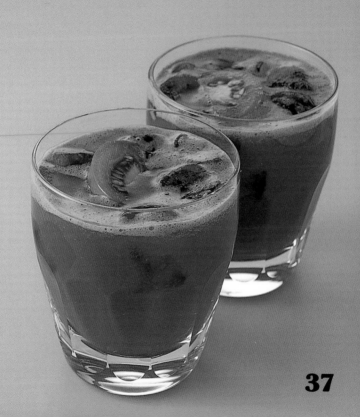

This juice combines celery and fennel, which help the body utilize magnesium and calcium to calm the nerves. Coupled with the sedative effect provided by lettuce, this drink is an ideal stressbuster.

green scene

50 g (2 oz) celery
50 g (2 oz) fennel
125 g (4 oz) Romaine
    lettuce
175 g (6 oz) pineapple
    chunks
1 teaspoon chopped
    tarragon

Juice all the ingredients then whizz in a blender with a couple of ice cubes. Serve in a tall glass and decorate with sprigs of tarragon, if liked.

Makes 200 ml (7 fl oz)

Nutritional values

- Kcals 128
- Carbohydrate 30 g
- Fat 1 g
- Vitamin A 3437 IU
- Vitamin C 68 mg
- Magnesium 47 mg

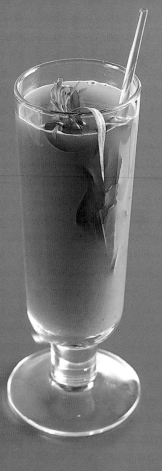

39

This is an absolute 'super juice'. It is a low-calorie, virtually fat-free burst of goodness, which will enliven your whole body and is great for lowering blood pressure, helping digestion, boosting the immune system and eliminating toxins. If your stress levels have risen to unhealthy heights, this is the best all-round juice, particularly if you are prone to migraines and nausea.

invigorate

2 oranges, peeled
½ lemon, peeled
1 cm (½ inch) cube fresh
   root ginger, chopped
100 g (3½ oz) beetroot
100 g (3½ oz) spinach
100 g (3½ oz) celery
100 g (3½ oz) carrot

Juice all the ingredients. Serve in a large glass decorated with orange zest curls, if liked.

Makes 600 ml (1 pint)

Nutritional values

- Kcals 286
- Carbohydrate 64 g
- Fat 1 g
- Vitamin A 34736 IU
- Vitamin C 510 mg
- Magnesium 164 mg
- Folic acid 310 mcg

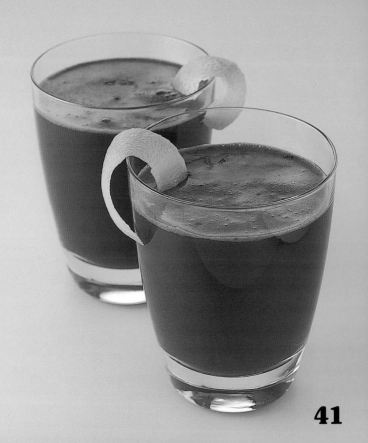

When you are really up against it and want a quick meal, you will find this smoothie very high in a number of nutrients and quick to prepare. If you want to make it even higher in magnesium and zinc, plus add a boost of vitamin B5, add one tablespoon of wheat germ, a raw egg or 100 ml (3½ fl oz) soya milk to the blend. This is also a good remedy if you are having trouble sleeping, as bananas and sunflower seeds are rich in tryptophan. This amino acid converts in the body to serotonin, a natural tranquilliser.

banana calmer

1 small banana, peeled
200 ml (7 fl oz) freshly
squeezed orange juice
25 g (1 oz) sunflower
seeds

Put the banana, orange juice and sunflower seeds into a blender with a few ice cubes and process. Serve in a large tumbler and decorate with some strawberry halves, if you like.
Makes 300 ml (½ pint)

Nutritional values

- Kcals 340
- Carbohydrate 74 g
- Fat 6.2 g
- Vitamin C 220 mg
- Magnesium 113 mg
- Tryptophan 85 mg

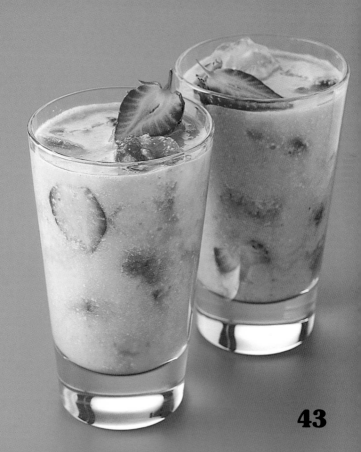

43

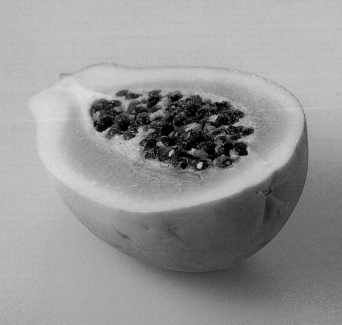

relax

When we are stressed, excess adrenalin makes our blood thicken, which can have a disastrous impact on health if the stress is prolonged. This smoothie is an excellent blood thinner and balancer, thanks to the avocado. Avocado is a good source of vitamin E and a highly effective antithrombin, which helps to prevent blood coagulation and causes dilation of the blood vessels, allowing the blood to flow more freely towards the heart. It is also vital to pituitary gland function, which ultimately regulates the adrenal glands.

go with the flow

150 g (5 oz) celery
25 g (1 oz) rocket
25 g (1 oz) watercress
1 apple
½ small avocado

Juice the celery, rocket, watercress and apple. Put the juice in a blender with the avocado and a couple of ice cubes and process until smooth. Serve immediately, decorated with a slice of lime, if liked.

Makes 200 ml (7 fl oz)

Nutritional values

- Kcals 267
- Carbohydrate 36.8 g
- Fat 15.9 g
- Vitamin C 35 mg
- Vitamin E 2.23 mg
- Magnesium 70 mg

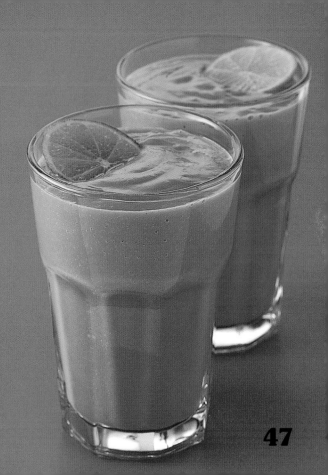

47

This naturally sweet juice is great if you have been overdoing it and feel a bit below par. Strawberries are a good source of vitamin C and have antiviral and antibiotic properties, while melon and cucumber both rehydrate and cleanse the system, which is essential for your liver, kidneys and adrenal glands.

cool juice

100 g (3½ oz)
   strawberries
75 g (3 oz) melon chunks
75 g (3 oz) cucumber

Juice the strawberries, melon and cucumber. Serve over ice in a tall glass, decorated with cucumber slices, if liked.
Makes 200 ml (7 fl oz)

Nutritional values

- Kcals 65
- Carbohydrate 14 g
- Fat 0.6 g
- Vitamin C 67 mg
- Magnesium 28 mg

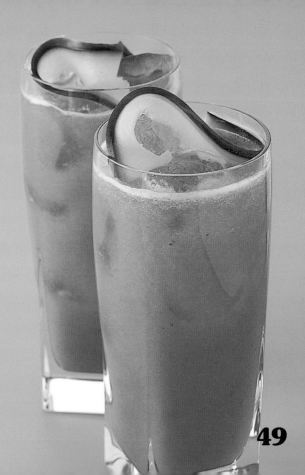

49

If you can't sleep because of the pressures in your life, a delicious smoothie at bedtime should do the trick. Soya milk and almonds are both very high in tryptophan. This is converted in the body into the brain chemical serotonin, which alleviates insomnia, calms nerves and helps to combat depression. This juice is also high in magnesium and vitamin C, making it an ideal booster for the adrenal glands and the immune system.

sleeping beauty

200 ml (7 fl oz) soya milk
2 kiwi fruits
**100 g (3½ oz) fresh or
  frozen hulled strawberries**
25 g (1 oz) flaked almonds

Put all the ingredients in a blender. If using fresh rather than frozen strawberries add a few ice cubes, then process until smooth. Pour into a glass and decorate with flaked almonds, if liked.

Makes 300 ml (½ pint)

Nutritional values

- Kcals 300
- Carbohydrate 36 g
- Fat 10.6 g
- Vitamin C 210 mg
- Magnesium 152 mg
- Tryptophan 171 mg

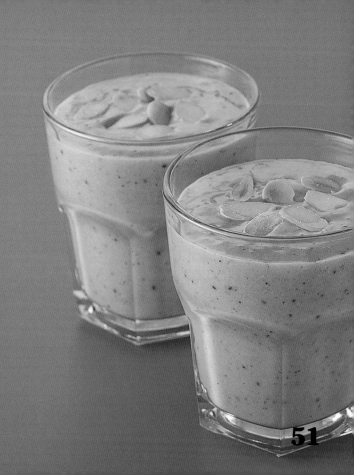

Lettuce and fennel are extremely calming ingredients. They contain calcium and magnesium, which are antispasmodic and produce feelings of calm, that may alleviate head pain and will certainly help in times of stress.

super soother

175 g (6 oz) lettuce
125 g (4 oz) fennel
½ lemon, peeled

Juice the lettuce, fennel and lemon and serve over ice. Decorate with slivers of lemon zest and lettuce or rocket leaves, if liked.

Makes 150 ml (¼ pint)

Nutritional values

- Kcals 72
- Carbohydrate 14 g
- Fat 0.4 g
- Vitamin A 4726 IU
- Vitamin C 67 mg
- Magnesium 32 mg

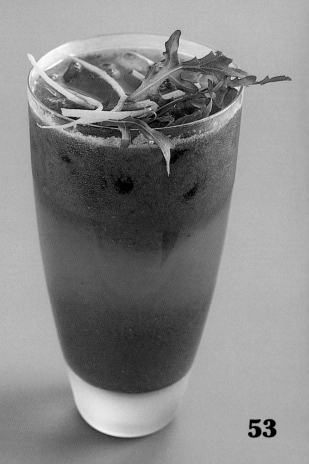

53

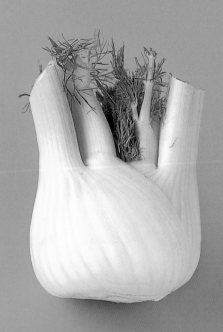

soothe

There are times when you are so busy and stressed that even going to buy fresh fruit is hard to fit into your schedule. Make sure you have these ingredients in your cupboard at all times so you can make yourself a quick energy fix at any time, day or night. Soya milk is highly nutritious and provides all the essential amino acids and is a great source of lecithin, which controls cholesterol. Both soya milk and sunflower seeds are high in tryptophan, which will increase the production of serotonin and aid restful sleep.

energy store

200 ml (7 fl oz) canned peaches in grape juice
100 ml (3½ fl oz) soya milk
15 g (½ oz) sunflower seeds

Put the peaches and their juice in a blender with the soya milk and sunflower seeds and process for about 20 seconds until smooth. Add a few ice cubes and blend again for about 10 seconds. Decorate with peach slices, if liked.
Makes 300 ml (½ pint)

Nutritional values

- Kcals 199
- Carbohydrate 39 g
- Fat 9 g
- Magnesium 73 mg
- Tryptophan 121 mg

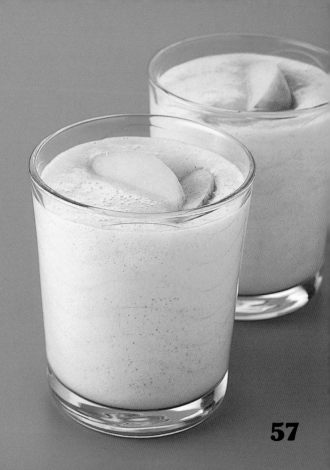

If you have been burning the candle at both ends and overloading your system with toxins, slow down and give your adrenal glands a welcome rest. This juice is packed with ingredients that will act as an effective tonic. Blackberries cleanse the blood and kiwi fruits are an excellent source of vitamin C, while the melon is full of beta-carotene and will help to rehydrate your entire system.

time out

100 g (3½ oz) cantaloupe melon cubes
100 g (3½ oz) fresh or frozen blackberries
2 kiwi fruits, unpeeled, halved

Juice the melon, blackberries and kiwi fruits, then put them in a blender and process with a couple of ice cubes. Pour into a glass and serve decorated with a few blackberries, if liked.

Makes 250 ml (8 fl oz)

Nutritional values

- Kcals 182
- Carbohydrate 42 g
- Fat 1 g
- Vitamin A 4194 IU
- Vitamin C 215 mg
- Magnesium 78 mg

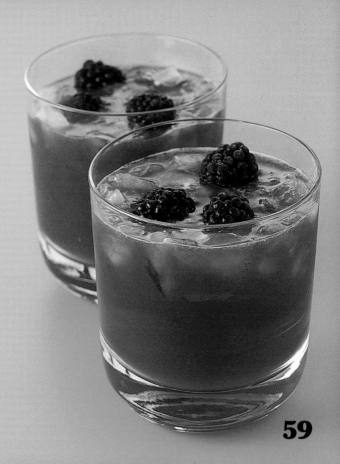

The vitamin C and potassium-rich ingredients in this juice help to lower blood pressure, which can be abnormally high as a result of leading a stressful life. If using the pomegranate seeds, stir in after juicing.

pressure point

250 g (8 oz) kiwi fruits
125 g (4 oz) cucumber
1 tablespoon pomegranate
seeds (optional)

Wash the kiwi fruits and cucumber but do not peel them, as both contain nutrients in their skins. Juice them, pour into a glass and serve with a slice of lime, if liked. If you wish, stir in a tablespoon of pomegranate seeds.

Makes 150 ml (¼ pint)

Nutritional values

- Kcals 168
- Carbohydrate 37 g
- Fat 0.9 g
- Vitamin C 250 mg
- Zinc 0.67 mg

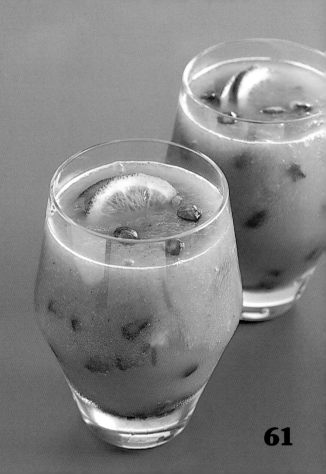

61

Stress weakens the immune system and reduces the body's ability to fight infection. It is therefore vital to replace the vitamin C that the adrenal glands use up, because vitamin C is the only vitamin that our bodies cannot store. So, give yourself a regular vitamin shot with this refreshing tangy juice. (Cold sores and lesions around the mouth indicate a vitamin C deficiency.)

pulpitation

1 large orange
½ grapefruit
1 lime

Peel all the fruit, leaving a little of the pith. Juice the fruit, then either serve over ice or, if you want a longer drink, dilute with an equal amount of sparkling mineral water. Decorate with curls of lime zest, if liked.

Makes 200 ml (7 fl oz)

Nutritional values

- Kcals 155
- Carbohydrate 40 g
- Fat 0.6 g
- Vitamin C 182 mg
- Zinc 4 mg
- Magnesium 38 mg

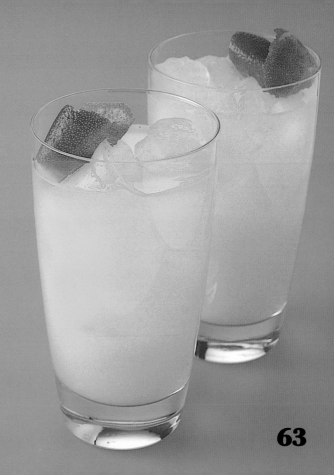

index

acknowledgements

The publisher would like to thank The Juicer Company for the loan of The Champion juicer and the Orange X citrus juicer (featured on pages 12 and 13).

The Juicer Company
28 Shambles
York
YO1 7LX
Tel: (01904) 541541
www.thejuicercompany.co.uk

Executive Editor Nicola Hill
Editor Sharon Ashman
Executive Art Editor Geoff Fennell
Designer Sue Michniewicz
Senior Production Controller Jo Sim
Photographer Stephen Conroy
Home Economist David Morgan
Stylist Angela Swaffield
All photographs © Octopus Publishing Group Ltd